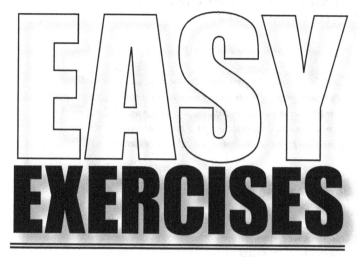

EASY EXERCISES

EFFORTLESS WAYS TO SLIP FITNESS INTO ANY ACTIVITY

JONATHAN KAMP

iUniverse LLC
Bloomington

EASY EXERCISES
EFFORTLESS WAYS TO SLIP FITNESS
INTO ANY ACTIVITY

iUniverse books may be ordered through booksellers or by contacting:

iUniverse LLC
1663 Liberty Drive
Bloomington, IN 47403
www.iuniverse.com
1-800-Authors (1-800-288-4677)

ISBN: 978-1-4917-3369-1 (sc)
ISBN: 978-1-4917-3370-7 (e)

Printed in the United States of America.

iUniverse rev. date: 05/13/2014

CONTENTS

For my sons, Niko and Dano, who suffered the long absences while I served my country.

Nothing in the world can take the place of persistence. Talent will not—nothing is more common than unsuccessful men with talent. Genius will not—unrewarded genius is almost a proverb. Education will not—the world is full of educated derelicts. Persistence and determination alone are omnipotent.

—Calvin Coolidge, 1872-1933

SAFETY FIRST

Always check with a doctor before beginning or renewing a fitness program. You are a dummy if you do not do this. If you let your body go for a lengthy period of time, you should not do anything that requires physical exertion without first checking with a doctor to see if your body can handle it. There are use-it-or-lose-it aspects to exercising, fitness, health, and dieting. Our bodies were meant to be exercised, and you should always be careful.

Next

Always warm up and stretch your body before any physical activity, and cool down and stretch your body *after* any physical activity. "Warm up" does not mean standing inside a warm room. It means moving your body around until your body temperature starts to rise. "Cool down" means taking time to stretch after you exercise—or after exercising, to walk at a speed lower than whatever speed you were walking at (for example).

If you have never stretched your body, think "specific yawning/stretching action," and then do it—yawn and stretch your arms over your head. The yawn-and-stretch action is the basic concept that you should apply to any muscles you plan to use. Google the phrase "flexibility exercises .pdf" (in Google Web or Images), or use similar search words in an online search engine, to find a chart with illustrations and captions for a person performing various body stretches. Print the chart, place it on a clipboard, and stretch your body.

Disclaimer

I've used the techniques covered in this book for decades. The idea for writing the book is to recommend that you look for ways to exercise smarter and wiser than you have in the past. You will be healthier if you do.

However, these methods do not replace advice from a personal fitness trainer or gym professional, namely because experts would most likely disagree with my methods. I do *not*, for example, recommend pushing yourself while exercising. I *do* recommend persisting with any past, present, and future exercise efforts – albeit at reduced levels.

To explain my position, I was forced to push myself to pass US Army fitness tests in the 80s and the 90s, as I was required by regulation to be fit at all times. With a heavy field schedule, finding time to exercise was often tough to do (there is much irony in this sentence, if you look for it). Looking back, though, this particular career pressure forced this book out of my head, as I racked my brain for innovative ways to exercise. So, all I'm doing is passing on to you the methods I developed—nothing more, nothing less.

Full Disclosure

I used to do things that your average civilian would consider to be dangerous. It would be trite and seem like bragging to regale you with tales of jogging in the desert after the first Persian Gulf War carrying an axe handle to ward off rabid dogs (I never had to hit one, thankfully; I love dogs). Or to tell you "war" stories about walking along ridgelines in training areas in Germany on moonless nights with night vision goggles covering my eyes. Actually, more often than not, the goggles were *not* covering my eyes—because the depth perception was iffy while wearing the goggles (I would take them off to keep from falling off a cliff). The point for not telling stories such as these is that I am **absolutely not** advising you to do anything dangerous. I am merely noting where my thought process comes from for this book. If you decide to start walking, hiking, or jogging more often after reading this book, please be a responsible adult and only do it in safe places. Please do not consider this book to be any sort of official exercise, fitness, medical, or dietary information—because that's not what it is.

Final Note (for this Safety First section)

You may have to spend some money to properly exercise. I talk about bicycles, home exercise equipment, and a little gadget called a Fitbit™ in this book—but none of those items are absolutely necessary to maintain fitness. However, a relatively expensive pair of running shoes— which means a *quality* pair of running shoes that will protect your feet in many ways—shoes that may also be used for walking—are essential equipment for many of the suggested methods in this book, and are well worth the investment.

PREFACE

The ideas I present in this book are methods I developed to assist me with exercising while I was in the Army. They are nothing special. I'm just like you—too much to do and not enough time. I have as much human nature as the average person on this planet:

o   I am lazy and do not enjoy lifting weights because it is hard work. Nobody actually likes work, do they?

o   I would prefer to go on vacation, sit by a swimming pool, and watch movies—rather than climb hills or do flutter kicks. I am not masochistic by any stretch of the imagination.

o   If I had my druthers, the words "exercise," "pain," and "drudgery" would always be used in the same sentence.

That being said, the compulsory fitness training I participated in while I was in the Army taught me that my body feels good immediately after certain types of physical activity—namely, cardio work (cardiovascular exercise that elevates my heart beat rate). Which may explain why I began looking for ways to interest myself in my own exercise programs: New ideas for ways to exercise would often appear in my head during or directly after exercising—creating an endless cycle of "exercise and thought," "thoughts about exercise," and so forth. I call it a "virtuous circle," and I probably talk about it too much in this book—but it exists, so there you have it.

If I were to rephrase the thought process for the above paragraph, I would say that I knew when I was on active duty that physical activity was good for me, otherwise the Army would not have constantly blathered about it while forcing me to do it. Couple that with the fact that I enjoyed being in shape *when* I was in shape—and you have this book full of ways exercise with ease.

Easy Exercises is also my way of saying "thank you" to the world for having my lifespan extended by way of the discipline that military life provides to a lucky few. And the cool part of this book is that after you read it, you may discover you don't need much effort or discipline to exercise—just your own good ideas.

EASE ON DOWN
THE ROAD

If you own a car, drive it somewhere.
It doesn't have to be a race car.
It can be a hoopty, truck, or motorcycle.
Park it in a safe place.
Walk back along a safe route.
To ensure you don't walk too far during your first attempt,
don't park it farther away than line of sight—
make sure you can still see it when you arrive home.

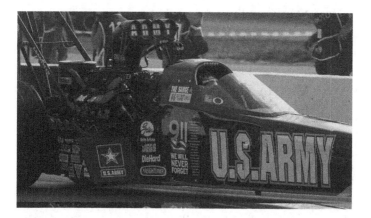

Essentially, that's all there is to this little trick (the photo caption above). Obviously, the farther away you park the car, the more exercise you will get, but don't do anything unsafe.

I've been doing similar things since the 1980s, and conceived of this chapter after parking my car seven or so miles away from my home and hoofing it back to my house. But please keep in mind that I noted in the safety notes that I walked a lot when I was in the Army—and have been walking in the woods in some fashion my entire adult life. If you park your car or truck a few football fields away from your house and walk back every day for the next year, you will have met the standard for this trick—although you obviously might want to walk farther than that someday.

The point for the concept is to place yourself in situations in which you *must* exercise—which is fairly easy to do.

You can, for example:

o   Jog home after work.

o   Nordic-walk to the mall.

o   Bicycle to work.

o   Walk to a bus stop farther down the line before boarding a bus to head downtown.

And, yes, I know that commuting and shopping distances are greater in the United States of America than in other regions of the world, and that everybody generally drives or takes public transportation everywhere. I *get that* every time I visit a military base or major city in the United States when people ask themselves, "Who's that well-dressed homeless dude walking around when he should be driving like the rest of us?"

At any rate, if you decide to start using human energy to transport yourself, always ensure that you walk or bike only in safe areas in your city or neck of the woods.

On that note, the correct way to describe this little trick is to call it "forced discipline," keeping in mind that labels are not as important as stopping what you are doing right now, and easing on down the road to park your vehicle somewhere to walk back.

Another Example

Here's another instance of forced discipline: Do some online research and shop around for an inexpensive, quality bicycle at eBay or a local garage sale. Once you're firmly gripping the handlebars, take it for a spin somewhere safe for ten minutes. Time the ride with a stopwatch or watch, and don't read the next paragraph until you get back.

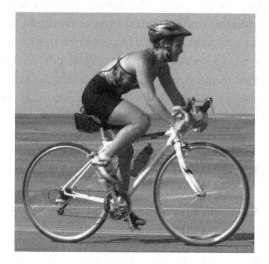

This is you whizzing by on a bicycle! OK, it's
obviously not *you*—but you get the idea.

The first ten minutes should be a breeze. The second ten minutes? Well, you have to ride your bike home, or you will be stuck in the middle of nowhere. And twenty minutes is the bare minimum for healthy heart rate elevation, so you just forced yourself to ride a bike for twenty minutes.

Sorry, I tricked you. Unless, of course, you read this paragraph before you took off on your bike.

Next Explanation

Buy a set of used golf clubs. Find someone who knows how to play. As long as you're not overly competitive, no one will care if you score 487 after 9 holes—because you just walked how far?

Again, it's just a matter of placing yourself in situations in which you must do some cardio work, and bear in mind that in many instances of newfound exercise methods, you will be using new muscles, and will be sore in fresh places around your body. I discovered this when a "golf pro" showed me correct posture and swinging methods, as the next day I was sore in places I did not know existed (I was unaware that muscles were located in those areas in my body).

Wise Guy Comment

If you still can't grasp the concept, here is one more example: Pay someone to fly you to the top of Mount Everest in a helicopter, and walk down. I doubt if this is physically possible, but if it is, as long as you don't trip and fall en route to the bottom—you can tell people you kinda/sorta "climbed (down) Mount Everest." Which would be a huge accomplishment you could use to regale people at cocktail parties, right? Right.

Satire aside, such a trek would aptly illustrate how to place yourself in a situation in which you must do something—or get off the pot. (Please do not attempt to do what I describe above; it was written entirely in jest.)

Carbon Footprints

If you need to explain the carbon footprint aspects of these techniques to someone, consider hoofing it or riding your bike back and forth to work for a couple of days. Which will allow you to point out all the fossil fuel you save, even though someone occasionally gives you a ride to a distant point specifically to allow you to walk or bike back.

Untold Safety Concerns

There are a huge number of safety concerns associated with traipsing off into the wilderness or through urban areas you are not familiar with. Please don't find yourself in a strange part of town, lost in the woods, or at Mount Everest basecamp contemplating doing something stupid (like climbing up).

And don't fall off any cliffs. It happens all the time to newbies. Even if you walk through a wooded, mountainous, or desert area near where you live—remember to stuff a map, compass, GPS navigation system, extra batteries, lots of water, a coat or poncho liner (never heard of one of those, have you?), and other safety and survival gear in your knapsack.

TWO BIRDS
ONE STONE

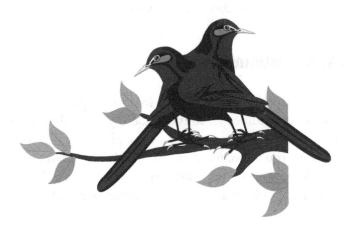

The obstacle that you avoid by
"killing two exercise birds with one stone"
is not a physical one.
Rather, it is the avoidance of the time/fatigue obstacle:
The one that causes most people to not exercise.

I probably came close to being discharged from the Army when I showed up for basic training at Fort Benning, Georgia, in the early 80s. I was out of shape, and the long runs during the first weeks winded me to the point that I could not keep up with the other recruits as they jogged in military formation. I was one of the guys you would see trailing the formation—barely making it—and I consistently failed the two-mile run portion of the fitness test.

Good Distractions

Lucky for me, there was an overweight guy who was having a worse time—and the drill sergeants were concentrating more on him than on me. He was not allowed to eat cake, and they forced salad on him at every meal in which salad was available (can't remember if they made him eat salad for breakfast). Plus, as you can imagine, they yelled at him a lot. The scenario sounds like a movie plot; I know.

Meanwhile, I had a battle-buddy who had been a long-distance runner in high school. He pointed out that the pain associated with jogging was in my head—that it was not a physical thing—and if I kept running, it would not kill me. He was right. I persisted. I began toughing out the runs and passing the fitness tests. Keep in mind that I was young; still a teenager.

Fast Forward

There is an immeasurable amount of institutional knowledge contained within the pages of military manuals. Some of the information is good, obviously accumulated from people who did things. Some of the guidance is sheer genius.

For example, according to a number of U.S. Army field manuals, it is preferable to avoid battlefield obstacles in training environments and in real life (something to do with the highly accurate artillery fire that may land on top of the concertina wire and other fortifications that form the obstacles).

If you apply the same logic to your life—it can solve a lot of problems.

Because That's What I Did

While on active duty in the 1990s, I used various methods to find time to exercise. For example, an Army officer drove past me once while I was jogging in a training area. He honked his truck horn, offered me a ride, but I declined because I had turned in my Humvee in a maintenance area and brought my running gear specifically to *avoid* vehicle rides.

To explain, I was jogging back to my office when I had the energy to do so. Rephrased (and as noted in the illustration caption above), I avoided the lack-of-time and fatigue obstacles that would have caused me to be too tired to exercise at the end of a long duty day.

That's it. That's how easy it is to find ways to "kill two birds with one stone" while looking for time to exercise.

More examples:

o   Combine an errand with a long walk—that's two things, right?

o   Walk or bicycle to work—two things are the commute and the exercise.

o   Walk your dog more often than you normally would: Dogs were domesticated by humans, so exercising your dog is a human responsibility. Plus, you'll get some fresh air and social interaction if you walk with neighbors and their dogs. (Hey! That's more than two things!)

o Sightseeing while bicycling along a safe path in your city. I live in a touristy area, and I was in the field so often when I was in the Army, and worked so much after I retired from active duty—that I was never able to enjoy the sights. I do now. On my mountain bike. Often.

And, yes, I know this chapter is a lot like the chapter before it. Which might explain the great lengths I went to dream up innovative ways to exercise over the years.

Final Thought (for This Chapter)

Don't let negative thought process invade your efforts. Taking the stairs instead of the elevator in a high-rise building is a cliché. Why not walk a few extra flights of stairs beyond your office floor—then back down again—to take full advantage of the concept of "taking the stairs instead of the elevator." Alternately, you could grab a clipboard and pencil before walking the length of your warehouse so people believe you are busy—because you are—as you check inventory or conduct building safety checks. When was the last time you looked at the expiration dates on every single fire extinguisher in your building, anyway? Heck, you might save lives with all your newfound energy.

Review or Comments

If you can think of a new "two birds one stone" exercise method, please feel free to write a review or comment describing your idea at Amazon.com or other online bookstore. Here's a place to take notes:

_____

_____

_____

_____

_____

_____

_____

TAKE IT EASY

We ran in combat boots and olive drab
fatigues when I first joined the Army;
kind of like this guy—no running shoes or fancy fitness uniforms.
But there's no reason to punish yourself like that.
As a matter of fact, just go on a long, leisurely walk.

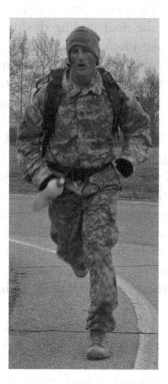

any people start jogging in January. Many people
stop jogging in January when they give up on
their New Year's Resolution to exercise. Pavement

pounding can be painful or even boring, if you're not used to it—and it takes time and effort to get back in shape.

Instead of choosing a date to begin or refresh an exercise program, why not do something easier *today*? The date you start an exercise program is not as important as persisting with the program. More to the point, place this book or your Kindle ebook reader on a table, get off the couch—and go on a walk right now. And make it a long one (call your doctor before you take off to make sure you're fit enough to go on a long walk).

If you're at the mall reading this on your tablet or smart phone, take a look around to make sure no one is watching—they might be reading the same book—then get up and walk the length of the mall, and then back to the other end. Since walking is a warm-up exercise, you don't need to stretch before you take off, but you should definitely stretch your leg muscles afterward. Again, Google the phrase "leg muscle stretches .pdf" (in Google Web or Images) to find a chart or illustrations/captions for a person performing various leg stretches—and stretch your legs.

After you've gone on the long walk, contemplate your situation. If you are or were a jogger who placed your exercise program on "pause"—it might be better to spend a year or so walking before you start jogging again. The way to examine the situation is with math:

o   If you walk once a week for a year, you've walked 52 more times than someone who quits jogging.

o   If you walk twice a week, you've walked 104 more times than the quitter.

o   Three times a week? 156 more times.

If you start jogging after you have walked for a year or so, it will be much easier because your legs will be accustomed to the exercise. If you end up walking long distance, you may even decide jogging is not necessary, as walking is a great exercise to maintain cardio.

Expand On Your Success

Similarly, if you lifted weights at some point in time, and then quit—look for the smallest set of dumbbells you can find. Look for the ones that are so small they look like rubber bicycle handlebar covers. Use those for days, weeks, months—maybe a year or more—doing all kinds of lifting exercises, to get your body ready for some heavy-duty weightlifting someday. Or not. Maybe just stick to light weights for the rest of your life because it's not as hard as power-lifting. Who wants to look like they're on steroids?

The same goes for floor exercises with gear such as medicine balls. Find the smallest, lightest medicine ball available, and bounce it off a brick wall for a year or so— before trying to throw one around that would knock the breath out of you.

Or do push-ups on your knees for years—then switch to real push-ups later.

DIY Inherently Better

Persistent exercising is more about wisdom than it is scientific health knowledge. The end result of a paid-for exercise program might be a person who does not stick with the program. I've watched this happen before at my gym. Obviously, this is not always the case; otherwise there would not be a fitness industry. Still, for those of us who are not as athletic as our local fitness trainer, it might be narrow-minded to assume we can perform at the trainer's pace, right?

Virtuous Circle

If you can determine ways to persist with exercise, an interesting aspect that evolves over time is the inherent addiction. For example, if you try walking once a week for a few months, you will feel the urge to walk more often. And, while you're walking or shortly thereafter, the cardio may force new exercise method ideas out of your head—creating a sort of virtuous circle.

Review or Comments

If while exercising, a new fitness idea appears in your head—don't thank me. But do feel free to tell me about the idea in a review or comment about this book at Amazon.com or other online bookstore. Here's a place to jot down your thoughts:

_____

_____

_____

_____

_____

_____

_____

CHANGE IT UP

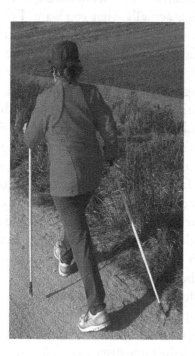

"It's sunny outside—let's go for a walk!"

Changing your normal exercise routine is similar to taking it easy on yourself. The only real difference is that you can make changes in either direction—harder or easier. Easier exercises obviously give your body a break, and can ward off injuries. "Harder" exercises do not need to be harder, in the sense that you do not need to suddenly take up running marathons as a hobby.

To make changes that seem hard, all you need to do is select a new exercise similar to one you are already doing—keeping in mind that this can make you sore in places you did not know existed (remember my recommendation to buy a set of used golf clubs).

And this is actually what you want. I've experienced the "undiscovered muscle group soreness" facet of trying to remain fit a number of times over the years, most recently with Nordic walking while searching for ways to continue jogging when I was in my 40s.

If you take a look at the illustration above, Nordic walking looks like someone walking with poles—because that's what it is! Someone walking with poles! If you're interested, search Amazon.com or your favorite sports store for "Nordic walking poles" in the Sports & Outdoors section (the poles will normally come with walking instructions). Once you understand how to walk and sort of drag and push-off with your poles, you may discover this relatively new walking technique exercises your entire body.

I didn't feel any difference in my leg muscles after my first long-distance Nordic walk, which meant I was either maintaining my leg fitness or giving it a break—because I was walking the same distances. But, wow, was I sore in my arms and other interesting places in my body.

Here are some ideas on how to make easy or hard changes to your exercise routines:

o   Changing exercise interval just means, for example, to take a two- or three-day break in between walks or runs, to alleviate pain or to preclude injury.

o   Alternately, take an entire month off from walking or running—to replace it with a new exercise. With cardio exercises, you can still maintain a healthy level of cardio fitness (your ability to jog or walk without becoming winded) by switching from jogging (for example) to long-distance walking, Nordic walking, hill climbing, hiking, bicycling, or gym treadmills and elliptical machines (that's the short list).

o In the gym you can change the type of weight machines you use to exercise different muscle groups. Changing the number of reps and sets you do is also an option. Gym professionals and personal fitness trainers can tell you exactly how many repetitions and sets of repetitions to do to eventually look like Arnold. But how about selecting the least amount of weight on a machine (the safest amount) and knocking out one set of 50 or 100 repetitions every gym visit? You won't look like Arnold when you're done, but you're exercising your muscles—and that's a good thing.

o For your home workouts, there is a plethora of new and interesting fitness equipment available at Amazon.com or any physical world sports store.

Review or Comments

If I haven't made my point for this chapter, I concluded over years and decades that changing my exercise routines facilitated lifelong exercise by allowing me to persist. Not sure if that would be considered another virtuous circle, but if you agree or disagree—feel free to write a review at Amazon.com or other online bookstore outlining your thoughts:

_____

_____

_____

_____

_____

_____

_____

PIECEMEAL

I f it's not obvious yet, I encourage myself to stay fit by not dreading my home workouts and everyday exercises. I make things easier. I place myself in situations in which I must exercise. I accomplish two things at once (don't know about you, but I get a huge sense of accomplishment when I get more stuff done).

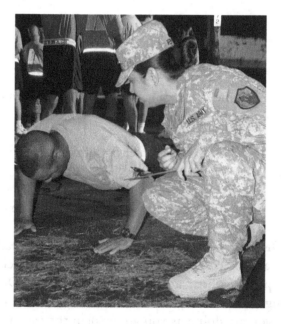

Hooah!

Put another way, I don't push myself too hard when I exercise, I suppose because there is no longer a regulation requirement to push myself (I'm no longer on active duty).

But many people push themselves to stay fit when there is no requirement—and I respect their choice. I just don't like doing it.

One way I avoid pushing myself is to spread out my sets. I do a little at a time throughout the day, which means I don't have anything to dread, because there's not that much to do.

Piecemeal Concept

Here's how it works:

o   Stop what you are doing.

o   Assume a standing position near a counter or doorknob.

o   Hold on to the counter or doorknob.

o   Do 5 or 10 leg lifts (lift a leg as high as you can, without straining it—and do it 5 or 10 times).

OK, you're done. Sit back down and keep reading. You can exercise more later. That's pretty much the concept: Do a little now. Do some more later. Do this throughout your day. It works best if you write down what you are doing as you go, or plan the exercises by writing them down and checking them off as you do them.

Agony of the Feet

Flutter kicks are an exercise in which you scissor-kick your legs while lying flat on your back with your hands under your behind. It's best done with no shoes; socks are OK, because they are nearly weightless in comparison to shoes. The reason the gentlemen in the illustration look like they are in pain, is probably because they're being forced to do 6,000 flutter kicks in one session—while wearing fins (6,000 might be an exaggeration).

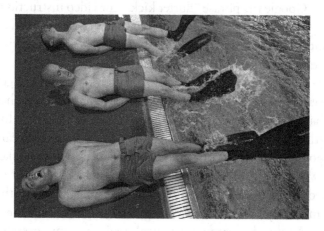

Flutter kicks are one of the easiest exercises known to womankind.
So easy, in fact—you can do them in bed, at the pool, wherever.
And you can cheat!

Since you probably don't have a Navy dive instructor or light infantry first sergeant yelling at you, you can do 5 or 10 flutter kicks—and then stop for a while. As a matter of fact, do 5 or 10 every weekend for the next year or so—or every day, if you're feeling "hooah"—keeping in mind that you can do as many as you want, as often as you like.

Flutter kicks work your abdominal muscles, and the reason I state in the photo caption that it's OK to cheat is because, technically, you are supposed to keep your legs straight, hold them a few inches off the floor, ground, gym mat, or your bed—and then scissor-kick them up to a 45-degree angle, then back down. But since you don't have the oversight I keep mentioning, doing perfect flutter kicks is not as important as moving your legs a number of times while they are off the ground to work your abdominal muscles.

Google the phrase "flutter kicks" for video instruction, if you need more instruction than that (Also note that flutter kicks are a variation of a swimming technique with the same name, but are totally different topics.)

My minimum is usually 100 flutter kicks before I get out of bed each morning, but there are many factors that change the number I do each day. For example, as of this writing, I'm doing 400 flutter kicks a day. A couple of years ago, when I was working and living in a place I did not like, I was doing 1,000 flutter kicks, either before I got out of bed, or piecemeal throughout my morning, which is the time of day I have the most energy for things like exercising.

Apply the same piecemeal logic to any exercise program – a little here, a little there, slowly increasing over time – and before you know it, you may be doing hundreds of repetitions of any particular exercise.

Piecemeal Cardio

The next question, of course, is whether piecemeal fitness works with cardio exercise? Absolutely. It's one of the tricks that perpetually skinny people use. Think of it like this: If someone moves around burning calories for 5 minutes out of every hour at their place of work, they meet the 20-minute minimum for healthy heart rate elevation if they only work 4 hours a day. They exceed the 20-minute minimum if they move around for 5 minutes every hour for 8 hours a day. You can't change the math involved.

In the Interim

The reason I would spend time telling you about piecemeal exercises is threefold: One, the A No. 1 reason most people do not exercise is because they are fatigued at the exact time they should be exercising. Two, the threat of having to run for an hour, or to take an hour or so out of one's day to go to the gym is what causes most people to "forget" to exercise. And, three, piecemeal exercise can prepare you for when you have more time to walk, jog, hike, mountain bike, and go to the gym.

Review or Comments

If you don't agree with the 45-degree angle portion of the flutter kick instruction, please feel free to vent by writing a review at Amazon.com or other online bookstore:

_____

_____

_____

_____

_____

DISGUISES

The US Army has an exercise program called "Master Fitness." The program I participated in the 1980s and 1990s covered ways to create exercise equipment out of items used in the field—essentially, how to use anything available to create exercise equipment. Sandbags, for example, could be tied to camouflage net poles and used as weight sets. The same sandbags could be used to add weight to a soldier's body during calisthenics, stacked to build weight benches, and so forth.

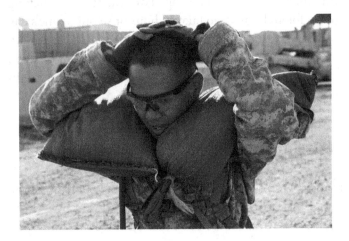

Nice shoulder pads!

So, this very short chapter is about how to adapt field expediency to your daily exercises and home workouts. You probably don't have many sandbags in your garage, unless you live on a floodplain—and that's not what I'm suggesting anyway (you don't need to build a bunch of field expedient exercise equipment).

What I'm asking you to do is to dream up ways to replicate traditional exercise methods with whatever. For instance, I worked in a mailroom at an overseas base a few moons ago, and when an annual shipment of 40 or so boxes of special-project printed material would arrive in my office, I would happily volunteer to move around the boxes with truck, dolly, and my body while people were deciding where to distribute the material. Sneaky, but I usually ended up sweating while moving the boxes, and would silently mouth the words "thank you" because the mailroom job could be sedentary at times.

If someone came along later and instructed me to move the boxes to a new location for better distribution, I would feign irritation—and then grin at any mirror that I happened to pass while moving the boxes. Of course, I never suggested new places to move the boxes around the base—that would have been underhanded.

With your particular situation, maybe you could volunteer to mow your neighbor's lawn or shovel their snow. They may squint at you a bit, but they'll probably let you do it. Easy stuff, right?

Review or Comments

If you volunteer to do somebody's job for them as a form of exercise, please let me know how it goes:

_____

_____

_____

DISTRACTIONS

This chapter is exclusively about distraction techniques, and is based on the US military tradition of singing cadence while running long distances in military formation—a technique arguably meant to divert service members' attention from the fact that they are participating in a gruelingly long jog.

It is guaranteed that at least one service member in any given running formation is slightly out of shape, and the Jody calls—the cadence singing—distracts her or him to the point that they forget about the run and finish with the group. Tricky, but it works.

Peer pressure is also in play. No one wants to be a service member trailing a formation a few hundred yards back. The cadences have much to do with getting into the whole "run" thing, too: Service members singing in one loud voice builds espri de corps.

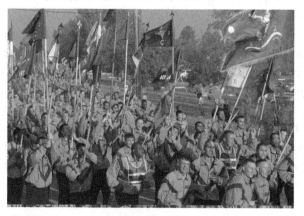

"Ain't no use in lookin' back; Jody's got your Cadillac!"

You can do the same thing. You can distract yourself from the discomfort or boredom associated with long-distance walking or running, and you don't need to jog down the street singing bawdy songs. You can form a neighborhood group that walks or jogs together, or just invite one other person to go with you for breathless conversation or the inherent competition of human companionship—both of which work like a charm as distraction techniques.

You could also pick an entirely new place to do your cardio work. Maybe somewhere with a view? Walking or jogging in a scenic area is a neat distraction, and it does not necessarily need to be a woodsy or deserty area to be interesting. Many cities around the world are building cool new, urbane walking and cycling paths smack-dab in the middle of their urban centers. Just don't be too distracted. Please watch where you are walking, jogging, or biking. There is a relatively recent urban myth about someone who was so distracted while walking that they tripped and fell into a snake pit. You will be fine while exercising, as long you do not ignore any of your five available senses.

If you opt for the gym as your exercise location, treadmills and stationary bicycles have built in diversion trays, if you've never noticed them (for books and magazines to read while exercising). Expand on that particular thought process, and maybe you can get away with plopping down a treadmill in your living room in front of your television to watch your favorite soaps or news as a distraction? I could not get away with something like this, but maybe you could.

Creativity

If you can dream up an exercise distraction technique that is more ingenious than US military Jody calls, please, by all means—feel free to write a review at Amazon.com or other online bookstore to let me know about your idea. This is not a challenge, of course—but I don't think you can (dream up one that is craftier):

_____

_____

_____

_____

_____

_____

_____

NAYSAYERS

The first person to slow you down when it's time to exercise will probably be you. But since I've told you how to eliminate a number of excuses, I would now like to point out that you may encounter exercise naysayers—people who get in your way, or who unintentionally try to slow you down when it's time to exercise.

Now you're saying, "What excuses? I haven't made any excuses!" Well, in the "Ease on Down the Road" chapter, I told you how to use other transportation means to place yourself in situations in which you must exercise—the forced discipline thing. In "Two Birds One Stone," I explained how to exercise and do something else at the same time—to remove the "I never have time to exercise" defense. If you've been too hard on yourself lately, I told you how to relax and "Take It Easy" for a while. In the "Change It Up" chapter, you can change exercise techniques to give yourself an additional break. With "Piecemeal," if you don't feel like doing everything at once, that's fine. You can use the "Disguises" technique to find even more time in your workday. And with "Distractions" you can divert your attention to something other than pavement pounding to distract you from the boredom or discomfort of said. Like I said, I've eliminated many of your excuses.

You're biggest problem once you start exercising again may turn out to be people who don't exercise. Let's say you wake up on a beautiful Saturday morning and see the potential for a long walk:

o It's Spring.

o The sky is blue.

o Every bush and tree in your city, town, or countryside has suddenly become bright green.

o The temperature is a little on the cool side because it's still morning—which is perfect because you will warm up once you start walking.

Nah. Your better half has different plans. He or she wants you to go shopping! And before you go, it's your turn to take out the trash! There are a number of other chores and projects to do around your home, and the best time to do them is right now! "There will be none of this crazy talk about 'exercise!' There are way too many things to do today, tomorrow, and the rest of your life! So get off this 'health nut' kick—*right*—*now*!"

I'm not saying that anyone has ever said anything like that to me, but I've heard other people discuss the mentality.

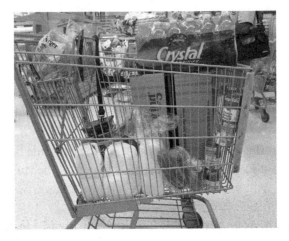

"Time to go shopping, Dear."

When it comes to exercise, one simple solution for naysayers is to try to avoid them. You can get up earlier than they do, or stay up later. You can try positive things like inviting them to exercise with you. You can go on an errand, but suddenly change your mind and drive to the park for a long walk through the park.

If all else fails, and you still get stuck with the shopping trip, park at the far end of the mall parking lot to extend your walking distance—and then sneak in a number of walks while you're in the mall.

You may have to apply large amounts of creativity to find the time to exercise these days, but whatever you do—never allow other people to slow you down.

Review or Comments

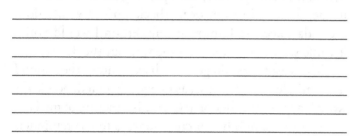

I have a rather large bag of tricks when it comes to naysayers. But if you have a technique that you think I'm not aware of, please tell other readers with an Amazon. com or other online bookstore review:

_____

_____

_____

_____

_____

_____

_____

SIMPLE REMINDERS

Reminders can be used with any exercise covered in this book—the idea being to develop cool, new exercise habits. If I could get away with parking my mountain bike inside, directly in front of my backdoor—I would do it every day, because I am relatively certain I would notice it while stumbling over it on the way out the door.

The reason I would go to such extremes—the reason I use reminders—is because, as previously noted, beside the word "lazy" in the dictionary there is a picture of my face.

Here are a number of creative ways to use reminders to facilitate exercise:

o   Park your car at an angle in your driveway to remind you to drive somewhere and walk back. The word-association reminder, of course, is that you are to do something "out of the ordinary." Parking your car or truck crooked—not straight within the edges of your driveway—would be considered, by some, to be "abnormal." If you're someone who already parks your car crooked, park it straight to cue you to drive somewhere and walk back. Until these exercise tricks catch on, driving a vehicle somewhere to park it and walk back would also be considered "out of the ordinary" or "abnormal."

o   Place your dumbbells on your kitchen or dining room table. Knock out a few reps while drinking your first cup of coffee as soon as you see them in the morning.

o   Set your walking shoes on the floor close to your front door (not somewhere where you will stumble over them, please). When you see them, say, "Oh, yeah," stop what you are doing, and go for a walk. If you think you don't have time to go on a short walk that might go long, there are at least 1,000 or so words in the chapters that precede this one that tell you how to find the time.

o   Program your alarm clock to visually or audibly remind you to do flutter kicks before you get out of bed each morning.

And So Forth

I use small wooden shelves throughout my home, placing various items on the shelves as reminders. I place my keys on the same shelf every time I enter my home, along with a pair of reflective trouser leg bands that I use to keep my right pant leg from getting tangled in my bicycle chain—specifically so I have the constant reminder to ride my bike to work. Like I said, I would prefer to park my bike in front of my backdoor—I just can't get away with it

Reminder about Naysayers

In the preceding chapter I talked about naysayers. These are the same people who will remove your reminders to put them somewhere else, because you are "messy."

HANG OUT

I wish I had more time to hang out at the gym. Actually, since you know me by now—what I meant to say was, I should exercise more when I'm at the gym. I'm in and out rather quickly when I go, as I usually only do a few upper body exercises on machines, a couple of sets on an abdominal machine, and some leg stretches. Maybe also some treadmill time, although I prefer long walks and mountain bike rides on scenic routes these days.

I do have two people in my life who rather consistently attempt to push me to do more, which leads to my rationale for doing less. Basically, you just have to join a gym or build one in your home and be consistent about minimally working out. You don't need to work out *hard*—because the math continues to point to the fact that if you show up at a gym and use one weight machine every time you visit—you're doing more than your average world citizen. You're definitely doing more than someone who joins a gym, works out too hard under the supervision of a personal fitness trainer—and then quits for the rest of her or his life because they are too sore to move a muscle after the one exercise session.

The basic idea is to create a gym attendance habit, even if you just stretch out and hang out at the juice bar. My ritual, for instance, is created by the expectation that I drive the two aforementioned people. I'm their ride. If you can produce a routine in which you show up at a gym, or walk into the extra bedroom you converted into a home gym—even it's just to watch television—you might be able to create a habit that causes you to exercise more. Just showing up is half the battle.

Gym Professionals Can Be Useful

If you opt for a gym membership, the safest way to learn to use weight machines is of course to ask for an equipment orientation by a gym professional or fitness trainer, keeping in mind that their general agenda is to push you to their limits.

Me? I sneak looks at the little instructional signs on machines—the signs and stickers with guys and gals with big muscles. But again note that I was taught how to assemble, disassemble, clean and maintain anti-personnel and anti-tank mines, and light and heavy machine guns when I was still a teenager—so I'm fairly good with figuring out mechanical things that I am unfamiliar with.

I.e., don't do anything dangerous because you can get hurt relatively easily with some of the machines. And again, I only use machines and weight sets that my body feels comfortable with. When I was younger, I felt uncomfortable while bench pressing weights to the point that I felt as though my body was not designed for such things, and I hated it. Today, it feels fine when I bench-press a weight bar or light weights.

Arnold

Arnold was not born with big muscles. Maybe he had genetic and other help, but his body shape still required years of hard work.

Your next mission, if you choose to accept it, is to not push yourself too hard in the gym, but ensure that you are still going to the gym years and decades from this point forward.

STRETCH IT

This chapter is about one back stretch. The point for dedicating an entire chapter to one stretch is merely to note that stretching makes exercising easier. That's it. I could almost leave it at that.

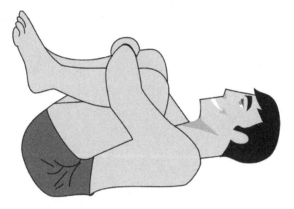

Are you out of shape because you are *wounded*?
Or are you "wounded" because you are out of shape?
No sarcasm intended.
I have lower back pain like the rest of the world.
(The reason this man is smiling is because
his back no longer hurts.)

Allow Me to Elaborate

If you're unfamiliar with stretching your muscles before and after exercising, Google the phrase "stretch your muscles.pdf" (in Google Web or Images) to find a chart with illustrations of a person performing various leg, back, and upper body stretches, with text instructions for each stretch. Print the chart, place it on a clipboard, and get busy.

Although stretching your muscles is obviously not a strengthening or cardiovascular exercise—it can extend your lifespan, as it increases your overall flexibility. In other words, stretching often can save you from tripping down the stairs because you are more nimble than you would be if you did not stretch.

Extend the thought process, and stretching your muscles is an exercise *multiplier*—as it facilitates exercise by preventing sports and fitness injuries. Which, of course, furthers your desire to exercise because you *can*, as you remain uninjured for longer periods of time. Another virtuous circle, if I ever saw one.

The Stretch (My Back Stretch)

I use the stretch in the above illustration to rise and shine each morning. If you can get your knee or knees anywhere close to your chest while counting to 50—you may be able to alleviate lower back pain. I, for example, try to pull my knees—one at a time—up to my face every morning before I get out of bed. And you can say I discovered this stretch by accident, but I prefer to believe it was a matter of persistence in my quest to maintain my cardio at an acceptable level (no huffing and puffing while walking up stairs, for example).

Long-story-short is that I've played racquetball for decades off and on, and while rekindling my game a few years ago, I immediately felt the effects of being old in my back. While doing my normal research for new back stretches—I Googled "back stretches .pdf"—and stumbled across the stretch in the illustration. The stretch caused my back to stop doing figurative cheetah flips, which was usually a sign that I was about to throw out my back—which would have precluded exercise for weeks after the injury.

This is not to suggest that this particular back stretch will solve your joint problems and suddenly allow you to exercise. Rather, it is to state that if you conduct some research into stretching your muscles and joints—concentrating on problem areas on your body—you may stumble across a stretch that will allow you to exercise more often. Like I did.

Review or Comments

If you solve an exercise problem with a muscle or joint stretch, please tell the world with a review at Amazon.com or other online bookstore:

_____

_____

_____

_____

_____

_____

_____

ANY DIET— ANYWHERE

Twice in my life, I have watched my weight "drop like a rock." Both times I scratched my head and wondered at this wonder of wonders. And then said, "Oh, yeah. I'm working a manual labor job and moving around all day. And sweating a lot." That, and whatever exercise activities I was doing at the time.

Without getting overly sciencey, both times were a matter of accidentally burning more calories than I was taking in. Which made me realize it's not that hard to do. Here's the short version:

o   Record calorie intake (food).

o   Record your calories burned (work or exercise).

o   Add a little of the aforementioned forced discipline.

o   Watch your weight drop like a rock—which, of course, facilitates exercise.

I know you're probably tired of hearing me talk about "virtuous circles," so I won't mention the fact that the above bullet comments form another one.

If you do decide to get sciencey, I recently bought a little device called a Fitbit™ to track my calorie-burning activities. The Fitbit™ comes with a web site that allows me to enter my calorie intake to compare the two numbers—a fairly simple arrangement for an old guy like me.

Full Disclosure

I like technology when it functions properly, which is to say I like electronics that do all the work for me, and that are not hard to set up. Thus, my full disclosure is that I have no connection to the company that manufactures Fitbit™. However, I have over the years purchased a number of similar devices, that for the life of me, I could not figure out how to make work (I'm not a teenager, aye).

I throw the Fitbit Zip ™ version I bought in my pocket so that it measures the calories I burn doing whatever cardio I choose. I note the specific calories for each portion of food I eat, entering the numbers at the Fitbit™ web site—then crunch the math.

If you use forced discipline to throw away all doughnut-like food in your home—or give it away as a means to making friends with one of your less friendly neighbors—and absolutely burn more calories than you take in—you can combine this method with any diet of your choosing, and lose weight. And subsequently exercise more. And write Amazon reviews about this book in which you recommend the author change the title of the book to "Virtuous Circles."

Review or Comments

Please write a review at Amazon.com or other online bookstore to let me know which diet you combine with this guidance:

_____

_____

_____

_____

_____

_____

_____

TIME OFF

This is probably the easiest of all techniques. Since vacations and weekends normally offer the most free time, all you need to do to conform to this chapter is adjust your priorities a bit. Plus it's fun, or at least I think it is. Heck, if I can find enough daily work hours to be a professional writer—and hold down day jobs—you can do the same thing with exercise.

Here are my suggestions for your next weekend, holiday, vacation or available off time:

o   Go on a walk on your next weekend.

o   Find a landmark on a map and walk to it on the next federal holiday.

o   Arrange for walking tours while you're on vacation.

o   Swim while you are on vacation.

o   Hike while you are on vacation.

o   Exercise before you go to work in the morning.

o   Arrange for a sabbatical specifically to find time to exercise.

o   Exercise if you become unemployed.

o   Exercise if you are a stay at home dad or mom.

o   Exercise during your breaks at work.

You know all my other tricks by now; e.g., walking or biking to work, and so forth. So, why not make your life more interesting by finally making that big trip to see the European Alps this summer—and take a few hikes.

Did you know you can call yourself a "mountain climber" by tackling a few "hills" over 2,000 feet (600 meters)? Arguably, 2,000 feet is the bare minimum elevation that may be referred to as a "mountain," although I don't recommend arguing about it until you've walked up one. And don't forget all the safety reminders about checking with your doctor before doing crazy stuff.

Alternately, if you're closer to Asia, what about flying to an exotic location such as The Beach. Which is, of course, the cool place on the planet where they filmed the movie of the same name. Phi Phi Islands in Thailand offer a number of interesting places to exercise, ranging from walking along the beach (ha), to swimming, snorkeling, and kayaking (watch out for riptides, aye). Rock climbing has also emerged as a relatively new sport on the islands, too.

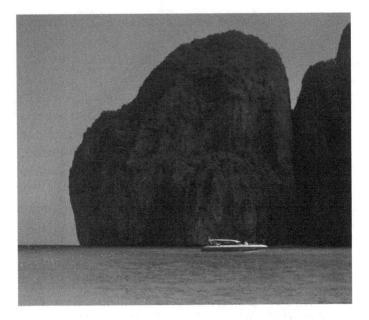

You don't have to scale the cliffs where they filmed "The Beach."
You can just walk along the beach, swim,
snorkel, and hike (in safe places).

The world is your exercise area, if you stop to think about it. If you're on a budget like I am, look around locally for interesting places to exercise. I have multiple ridge-lines near where I live that I have yet to explore. Many are well above 2,000 feet and go on for miles. I could hike to the top and just keep on walking.

MOTIVATION

I can't motivate you to exercise. You have to do it yourself. Hopefully, this book will inspire you somewhat, as I have pointed out numerous times that we are all different, and that traditional exercise may not be for everybody.

Understandably, my motivation while I was on active duty in the Army was "career." Which just means that a fast way to have *no* career in the Army is to fail a fitness test (a literal statement). I spent twenty-plus years in a near-constant state of slow-motion exercise panic, which caused me to constantly search for ways to make exercise more interesting specifically so that I would do it when I did not feel like it.

For example, while stationed in Germany in the 1990s I discovered a way to interest myself in my own running program. While jogging down a path beside the Danube River—the *Donau* in German—I noticed a river barge suddenly increasing speed. As I looked over at the barge, I heard its engine rumble louder and watched as its bow began to nose ahead of me. I was jogging at my normal slow pace, and although I had observed these flat boats many times, I had never really focused on their speed (because they were slow, too).

It's hard to see the ornery boat captain in
this image, but he's in there.

It may have been coincidence, but as I looked over at the boat captain, it seemed as though he was watching me with an evil grin. European river barges are elongated—some are monstrosities—with engine rooms and cabins at the rear of the boat. To me, it seemed as though the captain had been pacing me, and then suddenly increased speed to pass me.

Old ladies were jogging past me. Kids on tricycles were peddling past. Dogs were not chasing me because I was too slow to interest them. I was not about to let a hunk of metal pass me, too, so I sped up to pass the boat, and I remained ahead of it until a wooded area blocked my view of the boat.

The captain and I know who won the race at that point. And I used this new stumbled-upon technique many times after that, turning the tables on unsuspecting boat captains to pass them like they were standing still.

We all have to find our own pace, groove, comfort zone—and motivation. Some people may need a feisty competitor to force them to stick with a fitness program, or the social interaction, or whatever. Other people like to trail-run in secluded areas on the planet (that's me!). The boat captain thing was merely my way of converting something inherently boring—pavement pounding—into an interesting competition that motivated me to run faster. The method was especially helpful when I was out of shape from being in the field too much.

To some extent, the self-motivation I discovered with this particular method is the inspiration for writing this book. As I mentioned before, cardio exercise sometimes causes your brain to generate ideas by shifting it into overdrive via the extra electricity produced during heightened physical activity. Which means you should always have pen and paper, or cell or smart phone, available to record your thoughts when the ideas start popping out.

This usually happens during or after a long walk or run, and the entire process—exercise facilitating ideas for making your exercise and home workouts easier—becomes yet another virtuous circle (sorry).

EASY EXERCISES

Here's a list of the exercises, stretches, and other fitness techniques I've covered in this book. It's just a list, though—not in any particular order—other than kinda/sorta in the same order as the chapters of the book.

Please use your own creativity while Googling (Web/Images) the words and phrases in the list to find illustrations, instructions, and printable clipboard charts.

Don't forget to check with a doctor before attempting any of these activities—and remember to choose one—and do it today!

1. Warm up exercises.

2. Warm up stretches.

3. Cool down stretches.

4. Cool down exercises.

5. General stretching exercises.

6. Walking exercises.

7. Nordic walking.

8. Dog walking exercises.

9. Sightseeing walking exercises.

10. Mall walking.

11. Treadmill walking.

12. Hiking.

13. Hill climbing exercises.

14. Stair walking exercises.

15. Jogging.

16. Treadmill jogging.

17. Trail running.

18. Bicycling (don't forget your helmet!).

19. Mountain biking (on safe paths!).

20. Stationary bicycling.

21. Swimming.

22. Golfing.

23. Light weight lifting.

24. Knee push ups.

25. Elliptical machines.

26. Floor exercises.

27. Flutter kicks (don't forget: it's OK to cheat!).

28. Crunches.

29. Plank exercises.

30. Leg lifts.

31. Medicine ball exercises.

32. US military calisthenic exercises.

33. Sandbag exercises.

34. Desk raises; put your feet up on your desk and relax, it's OK to take a break every once in a while—just don't do it all the time.

AFTERWORD

I use a digital calendar to log my daily fitness activities as often as I can remember to do so. The assembled information makes a great searchable database for past activities, distances, weight, and so forth. Actually doing things is more important than keeping track of the information, though. I've probably forgotten to write down 25 or so percent of my activities over the last ten years, but it's not a big deal—because I know I was actually going on the walks, riding my bicycle, and doing the flutter kicks.

Try to record what you're doing as often as you think about it, because the information can help you brainstorm later for ideas. But always exercise first—think about it later—and don't forget to ask your doctor if you're healthy enough to exercise before beginning any activity.

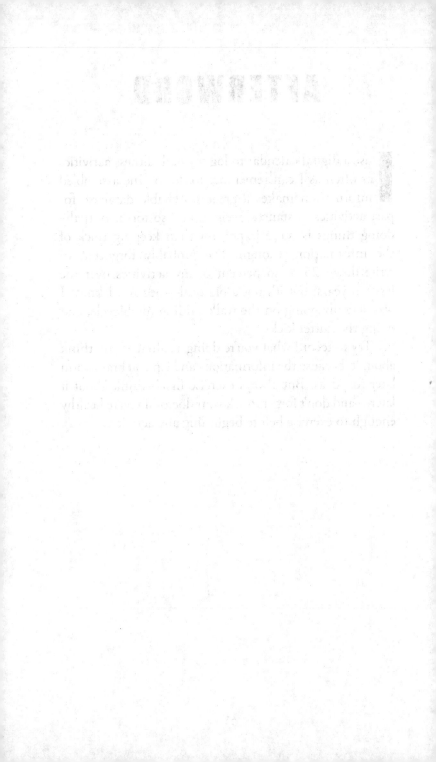

ACKNOWLEDGEMENTS

I would like to acknowledge the many people who sneak exercise into their daily activities (one of the many methods perpetually skinny people use to stay thin).

ABOUT THE AUTHOR

Jonathan Kamp is a freelance writer and former soldier. He was continuously employed by the US Army for 35 years—with over 30 years at overseas bases. As a stringer and infantryman on active duty he received two first place Department of the Army "Major General Keith L. Ware" journalism awards (1999/2000), and two first place Department of Defense "Thomas Jefferson" journalism awards (1999/2000). While studying for his BS in Communication Studies degree, he was awarded two President's Scholarships from the University of Maryland University College Europe (UMUC Europe) in Heidelberg, Germany—and completed the UMUC Excel (Portfolio) and Cooperative Education Programs as a freelance writer. He has written for up to two dollars a word. When he is not writing, he is traveling.

Scroll Creations Art—Jonathan Kamp interacts creatively with Warren Norcom and Scroll Creations Art at Etsy. Norcom's inspirational creations in wood may be found at ScrollCreations.com. His "STAY FIT" piece can serve as a constant reminder of the principles outlined in this book.

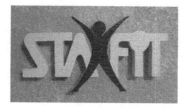